I0413981

MEDITERRANEAN DIET

30 DELICIOUS DESSERT RECIPES FOR A HEALTHY LIVING

© Copyright 2017 - All rights reserved.

The contents of this book may not be reproduced, duplicated or transmitted without direct written permission from the author.

Under no circumstances will any legal responsibility or blame be held against the publisher for any reparation, damages, or monetary loss due to the information herein, either directly or indirectly.

Legal Notice:

This book is copyright protected. This is only for personal use. You cannot amend, distribute, sell, use, quote or paraphrase any part or the content within this book without the consent of the author.

Disclaimer Notice:

Please note the information contained within this document is for educational and entertainment purposes only. Every attempt has been made to provide accurate, up to date and reliable complete information. No warranties of any kind are expressed or implied. Readers acknowledge that the author is not engaging in the rendering of legal, financial, medical or professional advice. The content of this book has been derived from various sources. Please consult a licensed professional before attempting any techniques outlined in this book.

By reading this document, the reader agrees that under no circumstances are is the author responsible for any losses, direct or indirect, which are incurred as a result of the use of information contained within this document, including, but not limited to, —errors, omissions, or inaccuracies.

TABLE OF CONTENTS

FREE GIFT

10 MOST EFECTIVE WEIGHT LOSS HACKS

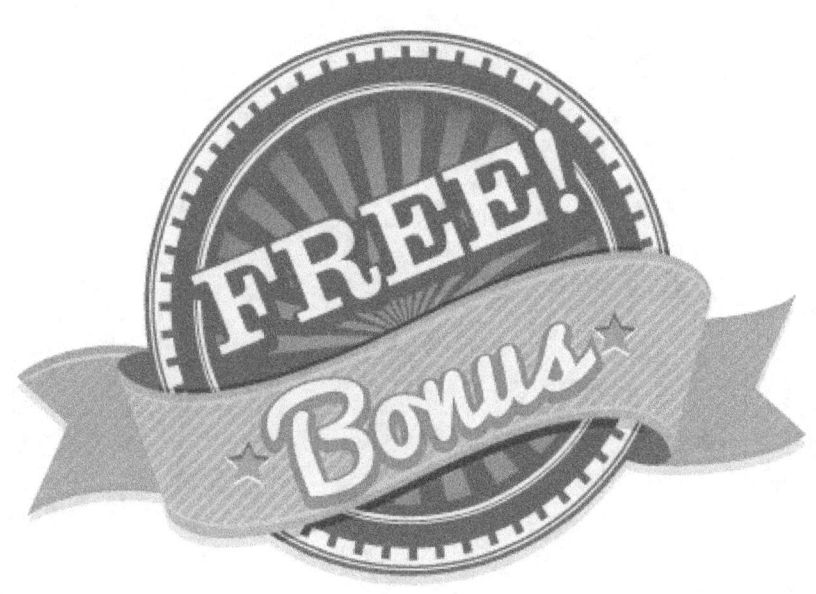

I WANT TO THANK YOU FOR DOWNLOADING THIS BOOK AND I WOULD LIKE TO OFFER YOU A FREE GIFT.

CLICK HERE TO GET ACCESS TO "THE 10 MOST EFFECTIVE WEIGHT LOSS HACKS"

OR FOLLOW THE LINK BELOW:

http://eepurl.com/cRXcDf

Introduction

I would like to thank you and congratulate you for purchasing this book.

Mediterranean diet has always been a very popular diet. Actually Mediterranean Diet is not a "diet", it is a culinary tradition that focuses mainly on eating fresh veggies and fruits, nuts, olive oil, whole grains and seafood. An occasional glass of Red Wine is also welcome. Mediterranean Diet just means: Eat Fresh, Whole Foods!

The Mediterranean diet focuses on eating more fish and less meat. It is very good for the heart. It has actually been observed in a study that the people who follow Mediterranean diet have a 30% lower risk of heart attack.

The Mediterranean diet improves the metabolism and help reduce cholesterol and blood pressure. Those who are suffering from high blood pressure, this is the perfect diet for you.

The Mediterranean diet focuses on eating the good type of fats like olive oil, seeds, nuts and avocado.

Summing up the Mediterranean diet:

- Eat More Fish
- Replace bad fats with good fats
- Reduce red meat consumption
- Eat lots of Veggies and Fruits
- Eat nuts daily
- Consume low fat dairy
- Eat Whole grains

This purpose of writing this cookbook is to provide you with some of the best quality Mediterranean diet Dessert recipes that are not only healthy but also delicious.

The book contains 30 Delicious Mediterranean diet recipes for a healthy living. The recipes in the book are easy to cook and does not require you to be a Master Chef.

These desserts will surely help you follow the Mediterranean diet in a better way and you will never be out of ideas to surprise yourself and your family with these delicious dessert recipes.

Strawberry-Banana

Smoothie

Servings: 2

Total Cook Time: 5 minutes

Nutrition: 340 Calories

 8 g Fat

 1 g Saturated Fat

 200 mg Sodium

 48 g carbohydrates

 4 g Fiber

 17 g Protein

Ingredients:

- 4 tbsp rolled oats

- 1 banana

- ¾ cup sliced strawberries

- 1¼ cup fat-free plain yogurt

- 1¼ cup skim milk

- 2 tbsp orange juice

- 1 tbsp flaxseed oil

- Ice cubes

Method:

1. Take a blender and blend milk, strawberries, yogurt, oats, orange juice, banana and flaxseed oil. Blend them until they become smooth.

2. Before serving, pour it over ice.

3. **Enjoy!**

Spice Cookies

Servings: 3 Dozen

Total Cook Time: 30 minutes+Overnight

Nutrition: 105 Calories

4.5 g Fat

38 mg Sodium

14.8 g Carbs

1 g Protein

Ingredients:

- ¾ cup extra-virgin olive oil

- ¼ cup molasses

- 1 cup granulated sugar

- 2 eggs

- 1 tsp vanilla extract

- 2 ¾ cups whole wheat pastry flour

- 1 ½ tsp baking soda

- ½ tsp salt

- 1 ½ tbsp ground cinnamon

- 1 ½ tbsp ground ginger

- 1 tsp mace

- 2 tsp ground cloves

- ¼ cup granulated sugar

Method:

1. Take granulated sugar, olive oil, eggs, molasses and vanilla extract in a large bowl and whisk them well.

2. Take another bowl and mix the baking soda, cinnamon, mace, ginger, flour, cloves and salt.

3. Now add the dry ingredients to the wet and stir them until they combine well. Now take the dough and cover it and refrigerate it overnight.

4. Heat up the oven to 350°F.

5. Line up 2 baking sheets with the parchment paper. Take the remaining 1/4 cup of granulated sugar and place it in a small bowl. Make 1.5 inch balls from the dough and roll them evenly in the granulated sugar.

6. Now place them on the baking sheets and bake them for about 10-13 minutes or wait till the tops of the balls crack. Now let the cookies cool down for 6-8 minutes on the baking sheets and then take them to a wire rack and let them cool completely there.

7. Serve and enjoy!

Special Peanut Butter

Chocolate Cookies

Servings: 24 cookies

Prep Time: 15 minutes

Cook Time: 10 minutes

Ingredients:

- 1 cup whole wheat flour

- 1 ¼ cups quick-cooking oats

- 1 tsp baking soda

- ½ tsp salt

- ½ cup peanut butter

- ⅓ cup olive oil

- ¼ cup granulated sugar

- ½ cup packed brown sugar

- 1 tsp vanilla extract

- 2 large eggs

- ⅔ cup mini semisweet chocolate chips

- 1 cup chopped nuts

Method:

1. Firstly, heat the oven to **350°F.**

2. Take a small bowl and mix oats, flour, baking soda and salt in it.

3. Now take a large mixing bowl and beat peanut butter, oil, vanilla extract and sugars in it until they become creamy. Add eggs one by one, keep beating properly after each addition. Gradually beat in the flour mixture.

4. Now stir in the nuts and the chocolate chips.

5. Take an ungreased baking sheet and drop onto it by rounded tablespoons.

6. Bake for about **9 to 10** minutes.

7. Cool on the baking sheets for about **2-3** minutes and remove to wire racks.

8. Serve and enjoy!

<u>Sauternes Cake</u>

Servings: 10

Total Cook Time: 1 hour 20 minutes

Nutrition: 280 Calories

16 g Fat

167 mg Sodium

26 g Carbs

5 g Protein

Ingredients:

- 5 eggs, separated, plus 2 egg whites

- ¾ cup sugar

- 1 tbsp combined orange, lime, and lemon zest

- 1 cup flour

- ½ tsp salt

- ½ cup Sauternes (or other sweet white wine)

- ½ cup plus 2 tablespoons extra-virgin olive oil

Method:

1. Preheat the oven to 375°F.

2. Take a 10 inch spring form pan and then grease it and also line it with a greased parchment paper.

3. Now take 1/2 cup of the sugar and the egg yolks and mix them and beat them until they become pale. Now add the zest to it.

4. Now fold in the salt and flour and then fold in the olive oil and Sauternes.

5. Take the remaining 1/4 cup sugar and the egg whites and beat them together until medium stiff peaks form. Now fold into the egg yolk mixture to form a smooth batter. Now pour the batter into the prepared pan.

6. Bake the cake for 20 minutes and then reduce the heat to 325°F and then bake for another 20-25 minutes, or until the toothpick comes out clean after being inserted into the center.

7. Now let the cake cool down for 20-25 minutes and then unmold.

8. Serve and Enjoy!

Raw Energy Squares

Servings: 36 squares

Prep Time: 5 minutes

Cook Time: 1 hour

Nutrition: 36 calories

　　　　4.5 g fats

　　　　1.5 mg sodium

　　　　8 g carbs

　　　　2 g protein

Ingredients:

- 2 cups pitted and chopped moist Medjool dates

- 2 cups raw cashews

- ½ cup raw almonds

- ¾ cup cocoa powder

- pinch sea salt

- ½ cup unsweetened shredded coconut

- 2 tbsp vanilla extract

- 3 tbsp cold water

Method:

1. Mix all the cashews, cocoa powder, almonds, chopped dates, and sea salt in a food processor. Pulse the ingredients together until the texture becomes coarse.

2. Now take the shredded coconut and add it and give it a quick pulse and then add the water and the vanilla, a little at a time while pulsing several times, until the mixture reaches a dry but moist dough consistency.

3. Now lastly scrape the dough into an 8*8 inch pan, make an even layer using a rubber spatula, and then chill it for about an hour or two before cutting into small squares.

Peanut Caramel Popcorn

Servings: 4

Cook Time: 20 Minutes

Nutrition: 430 Calories

      20 g Fat

      4 g Saturated Fat

      480 mg Sodium

      57 g Carbohydrates

      6 g Fiber

      9 g Protein

Ingredients:

- 2 tbsp peanut oil

- ½ cup popcorn kernels

- ½ tsp fine sea salt

- ¼ cup wildflower honey

- ¼ cup agave syrup

- ⅓ cup smooth peanut butter

- ⅓ cup peanuts, toasted and chopped

Method:

1. Take a heavy bottomed pot and heat it with peanut oil firstly. Now add the salt and the Popcorn Kernels. Now cover it partially.

2. Cover it completely when the popcorn starts popping. Now shake the pan till the popcorn slows down the popping. Remove the pan from the heat now.

3. Now take the agave syrup and honey in a pan and cook it for about 5 minutes. Take the peanut butter now and add it and whisk it until it is very well combined.

4. Take a bowl now and put all the popcorn into it. Now drizzle all the peanut caramel over it. Take the chopped peanuts and sprinkle them. Toss well.

5. Serve and Enjoy!

Parchment Baked Fruit

Servings: 4

Total Cook Time: 40 minutes

Nutrition: 235 Calories

2 g Fat

50 mg Sodium

56 g Carbs

7 g Fiber

4 g Protein

Ingredients:

- 1 peach, halved and sliced into quarters

- 1 mango, halved and sliced

- 4 apricots, halved and sliced into quarters

- 1 honeydew melon, chopped into large pieces

- Seeds of 1 pomegranate

- 4 cinnamon sticks

- 4 whole vanilla beans

- 4 tsp red wine

Method:

1. Heat up the oven to 400°F.

2. Now take 4 large sheets of the parchment paper. Take the apricots, pomegranate seeds, pear halves and melon pieces and divide them evenly among the four pieces of the parchment paper.

3. Cinnamon stick and vanilla bean should be used as the top on each fruit pile.

4. Now drizzle a teaspoon of red wine over each fruit pile.

5. Make a packet by folding over the edges of the parchment paper. Now seal them tightly.

6. Now bake until the fruit becomes tender (for around 18-20 minutes).

7. Cinnamon stick and vanilla bean must be removed before serving.

8. Enjoy!

French Honey Rye Cake

Servings: 1 Loaf

Total Cook Time: 45 minutes and overnight

Nutrition: 180 Calories

  1.5 g Fat

  0 g Saturated Fat

  50 mg Sodium

  41 g Carbs

  3 g Fiber

  3 g Protein

Ingredients:

- 2 ¼ cups whole rye (pumpernickel) flour

- 1 cup honey

- ⅓ cup ground almonds

- 1 tsp ground ginger

- ¼ tsp ground cloves

- ½ tsp cinnamon

- Grated rind of 1 lemon

- ½ tsp baking powder

- ¼ tsp baking soda

Method:

1. Heat up the oven to 350°F.

2. Take the honey and rye flour and mix them together. Let them stand overnight.

3. Now add all the ingredients and the spices and mix them thoroughly.

4. Take the dough and knead it for about 6 minutes and then spread the batter into a greased loaf pan.

5. Now bake it for about 35-40 minutes (or until a toothpick comes out clean).

6. Now let it cool for about 10 minutes after removing from the oven.

7. Remove from the pan and cool it thoroughly on a cooling rack.

Papaya and Mango After

Chop

Servings: 1 bowl

Prep Time: 10 minutes

Cook Time: 5 minutes

Nutrition: 100 calories

       1 g fat

       1 g saturated fat

       5 mg sodium

       0 mg cholesterol

       25g carbs

       3 g fiber

       20 g sugar

1 g protein

Ingredients:

¼ of a papaya or 1 peach, chopped into cubes

1 mango, skin peeled and chopped into cubes

1 tbsp coconut milk

½ tsp honey or maple syrup

1 tbsp chopped peanuts

Method:

1. Firstly, cut open the papaya and scoop out all the black seeds in the center. Take a serrated knife and slice off the skin of the papaya.

2. Slice it lengthwise into quarters and then chop into bite-size cubes.

3. Now take a knife or peeler and then peel off your Mango. Chop the mango chunks into some bit sized cubes.

4. Now place the fruits in a bowl and then drizzle the honey, coconut milk, and peanuts over the fruits. Stir to coat.

5. Serve it immediately or chilled. **Yum!**

Tip!

Change the fruits according to the season and choice.

Carrot Cake

Servings: 10

Total Cook Time: 1 hour

Nutrition: 625 Calories

27 g Total Fat

5 g Saturated Fat

270 mg Sodium

93 g Carbs

4 g Fiber

10 g Protein

Ingredients:

- For the cake:

- 2 cups grated carrot

- 2 cups self-rising whole wheat flour

- 1 teaspoon baking powder

- ½ teaspoon baking soda

- 1 cup dried fruit

- ½ cup chopped walnuts

- 1 cup soft brown sugar

- 1 teaspoon mixed spice

- Pinch of salt

- ¾ cup walnut oil

- 2 eggs, beaten

- For the icing:

- 8 ounces neufchatel cheese, softened

- 3 cups unrefined icing sugar

- Scant ½ cup cultured buttermilk

Method:

Making the Cake:

1. First of all, heat up the oven to 350°F.

2. Take the carrots, baking powder, flour, baking soda, brown sugar, dried fruit, salt and the spice and mix them all in a large bowl.

3. Now add eggs and walnut oil and beat the mixture together.

4. Take an 8 inch pan and bake in it at 330°F for around 55-60 minutes.

5. If the tester comes out clean, remove it from the oven.

6. Before icing, let the cake cool down.

For the Icing:

1. Take the icing sugar and neufchatel cheese and then beat them together.

2. Now stir in the buttermilk till the mixture becomes soft and smooth.

Black Olive

Servings: 16

Prep Time: 1 hour

Nutrition: 220 Calories

       10 g Fats

       2 g Saturated Fat

       190 mg Sodium

       33 g carbohydrates

       3 g Fiber

       4g Protein

Ingredients:

2 cups whole wheat pastry flour

1 tsp baking powder

1 tsp baking soda

2 tsp ground cardamom

1 tsp ground cloves

1 tsp ground cinnamon

3 eggs

½ cup extra-virgin olive oil

1 cup plain Greek yogurt

3 tbsp pomegranate molasses

1 ½ cups or 1 can (6 oz.) pitted black olives, chopped

Grated zest and juice from 1 orange

½ cup currants

1 cup crystallized ginger, diced

2 tbsp fennel seeds

1 ½ cups of confectioners sugar (for glaze)

Method:

1. Preheat the oven to **350°F.** Take a **9 inch** cake pan and then grease it. Now cover the pan with a circle of parchment paper, and then grease the paper.

2. Now combine the flour, baking powder and soda, cardamom, cinnamon, and cloves in a large bowl and then blend it with a whisk. Set it aside.

3. Now take a mixing bowl and mix the olive oil, eggs, yogurt and **2 tbsp** of the pomegranate molasses and whisk it until it gets smooth. Now stir in the dry ingredients. Fold in the orange zest, olives, ginger, currants and fennel seeds. Stir it until it gets smooth.

4. Now take the batter and spoon it into the cake pan and bake it for around **40** minutes, or until the cake becomes lightly browned and a toothpick comes out clean if it is inserted in the center. Now transfer the cake to a rack for cooling.

5. Run a knife around the edges of the cake when it has cooled slightly but is still a little bit warm. Now take a flat plate and put it on top of the cake and then flip the cake on to the plate. Now cover the cake with a serving plate and flip it into the plate again.

6. Now combine **1** tablespoon of pomegranate molasses and two tablespoons of the orange juice in a small saucepan and then bring it just to the simmer. Now cook it for about **1 minute** after adding the sugar, whisking to form a smooth glaze. Now pour the glaze over the cake.

7. Serve it warm or let it cool. **Enjoy!**

Bean Brownies

Servings: 16 Brownies

Prep Time: 10 minutes

Cook Time: 50 minutes

Nutrition: 147 calories

>   8 g fat

>   2 g saturated fat

>   99 mg sodium

>   20 g carbs

>   3 g fiber

>   3 g protein

Ingredients:

- Nonstick cooking spray

- One (15-ounce) can black beans, 0 salt added, rinsed and drained (or 1¾ cup cooked)

- ½ cup honey, agave nectar, or maple syrup

- ½ cup unsweetened cocoa powder

- 2 tbsp chia seeds

- 1 tsp pure vanilla extract

- 3 tbsp expeller-pressed canola oil

- ½ tsp of baking powder

- ½ cup dairy-free, dark-chocolate chips

- ½ cup chopped walnuts or pecans

Method:

1. Firstly, heat the oven to **350°F.** Take a **8*8** inch baking dish and spray it with the non stick cooking spray.

2. Take a food processor or blender and put the honey, black beans, cocoa powder, vanilla, chia seeds, baking powder and canola oil. Process them until they become smooth. If required, scrape down the sides halfway through blending.

3. Take the baking dish that you prepared earlier and pour the batter into it.

4. Now take the walnuts and chocolate chips and sprinkle them evenly across the top of your brownies.

5. Now bake for about **46 to 50** minutes. Wait until the brownies become firm and their edges pull away from the side of the pan.

6. Half way through baking, put a little piece of aluminum foil over the brownies to prevent the nuts from getting too brown.

7. Let it cool for a few minutes, and then slice it into **16** square pieces.

Baked Fruit

Servings: 4

Cook Time: 30 Minutes

Nutrition: 230 Calories

      2 g Total Fat

      50 mg Sodium

      56 g Carbohydrates

      7 g Fiber

      4 g Protein

Ingredients:

- 1 peach, halved and sliced into quarters

- 1 mango, halved and sliced

- 4 apricots, halved and sliced into quarters

- 1 honeydew melon, chopped into large pieces

- Seeds of 1 pomegranate

- 4 cinnamon sticks

- 4 whole vanilla beans

- 4 teaspoons red wine

Method:

1. Firstly, Heat up the oven to **400°F.**

2. Take four large sheets of parchment paper and tear them off.

3. Take the apricots, pomegranate seeds, pear halves and melon pieces and distribute them evenly among the pieces of parchment.

4. Put **1** Cinnamon Stick and **1** Vanilla Bean on top of each fruit pile and also drizzle **1** tsp of Red Wine on each of the fruit pile.

5. Form a packet by folding over the edges of the parchment paper. Seal it tightly.

6. Now bake for about **20** minutes.

7. Now before you serve, remove the Cinnamon Stick and Vanilla Bean.

8. Enjoy!

Tip!

Experiment with different fruits to add more flavor to the dish. Go with your favorite fruits or with the seasonal ones.

Sweet Pumpkin Soufflés

Servings: 4

Prep Time: 35 minutes

Nutrition: 267 calories

   7 g total fat

   2 g saturated fat

   277 mg cholesterol

   169 mg sodium

   42 g carbohydrates

   1 g fiber

   10 g protein

Ingredients:

- Sugar for soufflé dishes

- 6 egg whites, room temperature

- ¾ tsp cream of tartar

- ½ cup sugar

- 6 egg yolks

- ½ cup canned pumpkin

- ½ tsp pumpkin pie spice

Method:

1. Preheat the oven to **375°F.** Now coat four lightly greased **8** ounce soufflé dishes evenly with sugar. Now place them in a baking pan.

2. Take a mixer bowl with a whisk attachments and beat the egg whites and cream of tartar on high speed until foamy. Keep beating constantly, add **half** cup sugar, **two** tbsp at a time, beating after each addition until the sugar is dissolved adding the next time. Keep beating until the whites become glossy and stand in the soft peaks.

3. Take a separate bowl and beat the egg yolks on high speed until they become thick and lemon colored. Then fold it in pumpkin and pie spice. Now fold the yolk mixture into whites until no streaks of the white remain. Pour evenly into the soufflé dishes.

4. Now take the pan with the soufflé dishes and place it on a rack in the middle of the

oven. Now take very hot water and pour it into the pan to within half inch of the top of the dishes and then bake until the soufflés become puffy and delicately browned, around **16-20** minutes.

5. Serve it immediately. **Enjoy!**

Sultana Yogurt Cake

Servings: 6

Total Cook Time: 1 hour 30 minutes

Nutrition: 280 calories

   7 g fat

   2 g saturated fat

   40 g carbohydrates

   90 mg sodium

   2 g fiber

   16 g protein

Ingredients:

- ¼ cup sultanas or golden raisins, roughly chopped

- Muscat or sherry

- 5 eggs, yolks and whites separated

- ⅓ cup sugar

- 3 tbsp honey

- ¾ cups white whole wheat flour, sifted

- 17 ounces plain Greek yogurt (about 2 cups)

- Zest and juice of 1 lemon

- 1 tbsp olive oil

Method:

1. Firstly, grease an **8** inch spring form cake pan and also heat the oven to **350°F.**

2. Now take a small bowl and cover all the sultanas in muscat and put them aside and let them soak for about **10 minutes.** Now drain the sultanas and set them aside.

3. Take sugar, egg yolks and honey and beat them with a electric mixer until they become thick and creamy.   Now add the sultanas, flour, yogurt, juice, zest and oil. Mix them on low until they are well combined.

4. Take another bowl, combine the egg whites until they become stiff, then take a spoonful of the whipped egg whites and stir them into the yogurt mixture to slacken it.

5. Now gently fold all the remaining egg whites. Make sure that the mixture is light and airy.

6. Now bake for **55 to 60** minutes after pouring it into the cake pan. The top will become brown and the cake will puff up like a soufflé. Now remove it from the oven and let it cool in the pan. Use a knife to loosen the cake once it starts to subside away from the edges of the pan.

7. Now **unclip** the spring form pan and allow the cake to cool.

8. Serve and enjoy!

Avocado Banana Blue

Berry Bang

Servings: 2

Cook time: 5 minutes

Nutrition: 250 Calories

13 g Fat

1.5 g Saturated fat

10 mg Sodium

37 g Carbohydrate

15 g fiber

4 g Protein

Ingredients:

- 1 frozen banana, peeled and cut in chunks

- 2 ripe avocados, seeded, peeled and quartered*

- 2 cups fresh or frozen berries (use your favourite combinations of blackberries, blueberries, raspberries or strawberries)

- Ice water, as needed

- Agave or maple syrup, to taste

Method:

1. Firstly, take a blender place frozen banana chunks, berries, and avocado and puree until smooth by adding a ¼ cup of ice water at a time as needed to achieve desired consistency.

2. Now, taste it and if desired sweeten it with agave or maple syrup.

3. Pour it into tall glasses, leaving behind any berry seeds at bottom of blender.

4. Serve chilled.

Spiced Medjool Date And

Walnut Brownies

Servings: 16

Cook time: 1 hour 5 minutes

Nutrition: 165 calories

> 7 g total fat
>
> 1 g saturated fat
>
> 63 mg sodium
>
> 26 g carbohydrates
>
> 3.5 g fiber
>
> 4 g protein

Ingredients:

- 1 cup whole wheat flour

- ½ cup cocoa powder

- 2 teaspoons ground cinnamon

- 1 teaspoon baking powder

- ¼ teaspoon sea salt

- ½ cup coarsely chopped walnuts

- 16 Medjool dates, pitted

- 2 eggs

- 4 egg whites (about ¼ cup)

- ¼ cup olive oil

- 1 teaspoon pure vanilla extract

Method:

1. Firstly, preheat the oven to **350° F.**

2. Take a medium size bowl and whisk flour, cocoa powder, cinnamon, baking powder, and salt in it. Stir it in walnuts and put it aside.

3. Combine dates, eggs, eggs whites, oil and vanilla in a food processor. Mix them well until combine and smooth.

4. Now gradually mix wet ingredients into dry ingredients, until just combined. Take care that you do not over mix it. (Mixture will be very thick)

5. Take an **8×8 –inch** baking pan spray sides of it with cooking spray. Now pour batter into pan and place into oven. Bake it for about **16** minutes or until a toothpick inserted into the center comes out clean.

6. Now take out the pan from the oven and allow brownies to cool to room temperature for about **30** minutes.

7. Then, loosen brownie and turn slab out onto a cutting board or platter. Cut it into **16** pieces, wrap it with plastic wrap and place it in refrigerator for a night.

8. Leftovers may be kept refrigerated in a resealable container for up to **2** days.

9. Serve and **enjoy the sweetness.**

Sfouf Bi Dibs

Servings: 20

Cook time: 55 minutes

Nutrition: 340 Calories

        12 g Fat

        1 g Saturated fat

        45 mg Sodium

        50 g Carbohydrate

        2 g fiber

        5 g Protein

Ingredients:

- 3 cups semolina flour
- 3 cups white whole wheat flour

- 2 teaspoons baking powder
- 2 teaspoons ground anise seed
- 1 teaspoon vanilla
- 1 cup canola oil
- 1½ cups water
- 1½ cups carob molasses
- 2 tablespoons tahini (sesame paste)
- Sesame seeds, slivered almonds or pine nuts to garnish

Method:

1. Firstly, preheat the oven to 350 F.

2. Mix semolina, whole wheat flour, baking powder, anise seed, and vanilla in a bowl. Add oil in it and stir to make a paste.

3. Mix water and carob molasses gradually to the flour with the help of an electric cake mixer.

4. Use tahini and pour batter in it to grease the baking dish. Taking care that it is flat and even.

5. Sprinkle sesame, pine nuts, or almonds on it.

6. Bake it for about 30 minutes or until it turns golden-brown.

7. Cool it for 15 minutes and cut it in pieces as you do for your brownies.

8. Serve and enjoy.

Sauteed Bosc Pears With

Walnuts

Servings: 6

Cook time: 30 minutes

Nutrition: 220 Calories

       10 g Fat

       3 g Saturated Fat

       35 mg Sodium

       31g Carbohydrate

       6 g Fiber

       2 g Protein

*(not including ice cream and yogurt)

Ingredients:

- 2 tablespoons salted butter
- ¼ teaspoon cinnamon
- ¼ teaspoon ground nutmeg
- ¼ teaspoon ground allspice
- 6 Bosc pears, peeled, cored and quartered
- Juice of ½ lemon
- ½ cup chopped, toasted walnuts

Method:

1. Firstly, for preparing pears, melt the butter in a large skillet over medium heat.

2. Then, stir it in spices and cook it for about 30 seconds or until aromatic.

3. Now, add pears to it and cook it for about 15 minutes or until it becomes tender.

4. Keep stirring it frequently in lemon juice.

5. Decorate it's top with walnuts. Serve with yogurt or cheese.

6. Enjoy.

Greek Yogurt With Honey

Macerated Citrus and

Medjool Dates

Servings: 2

Cook time: 10 Minutes

Nutrition: 380 Calories

       0 g Fat

       0 g Saturated Fat

       60 mg Sodium

       89 g Carbohydrates

       11 g Fiber

       16 g Protein

Ingredients:

- 1 cup plain, nonfat Greek yogurt

- 2 medium oranges

- 4 to 6 Medjool Dates, pitted and chopped

- 2 tablespoons honey

- 2 tablespoons chopped pistachio kernels or pomegranate arils (optional)

Method:

1. Take a small bowl and place yogurt in it.

2. Take off the peel from the orange by carefully cutting off each end and then sliding down the sides.

3. Squeeze out the juice from the peels over yogurt.

4. Now, first slice the fruit over circles and then in half to form semicircles.

5. **Carefully** arrange them over the yogurt.

6. Now drizzle it with honey and sprinkle with dates and pistachios.

7. Refrigerate it few hours before you serve it so that the dish macerate.

8. Serve and **enjoy.**

Dried Figs

Servings: 4

Serving Size: 2 figs

Cook time: 15 Minutes

Nutrition: 142 Calories

8 g Fat

1 g Saturated Fat

21 mg Sodium

17 g Carbohydrates

2 g Fiber

4 g Protein

Ingredients:

- 8 dried figs

- ¼ cup part skim ricotta cheese

- 16 walnut halves

- 1 tablespoon honey

Method:

1. Firstly, toast the walnuts in a dry skillet over a medium- high heat for about 2 minutes till they start fragmenting.

2. Then put it aside to cool down.

3. Now make a small indentation into the cut side of each fig half with the help of a small spoon or your finger.

4. Carefully, put a ½ teaspoon of the ricotta cheese into each individual piece of the fig and beautifully top it with a walnut half.

5. Finally, drizzle each fig with honey.

6. Serve and **enjoy.**

Date Porcupines

Servings: 36

Cook time: 25 minutes

Nutrition: 65 calories

       1 g fat

       5 mg sodium

       8 g carbohydrate

       1 g protein

Ingredients:

- 2 eggs
- 1 tablespoon extra-virgin olive oil
- 1 teaspoon vanilla

- 1 cup pitted, chopped Medjool dates, (about 10)

- 1 cup chopped walnuts

- ¾ cup all-purpose flour

- ½ teaspoon salt

- 1 cup sweetened shredded coconut

Method:

1. Firstly, preheat the oven to 350 F. Now lightly grease a large baking sheet.

2. Take a large bowl, beat eggs well in it and add the olive oil and vanilla in it. Now fold in the dates and walnuts.

3. Sift the flour and salt together and then gradually add date and egg mixture in it. Mix everything well.

4. Now, start forming mixture into small balls (about   tablespoon each) and roll them in coconut.

5. Arrange them on a baking sheet and bake them for about 12-15 minutes, until the coconut began to turn golden. Now transfer it to a wire rack to cool completely.

6. Serve and **enjoy.**

Chocolate Mousse

Servings: 6

Cook time: 20 Minutes

Nutrition: 490 Calories

> 37 g Fat
>
> 12 g Saturated Fat
>
> 80 mg Sodium
>
> 30 g Carbohydrates
>
> 4 g Fiber
>
> 8 g Protein

Ingredients:

- 9½ ounces extra bitter dark chocolate
- ⅔ cup extra virgin olive oil

- 3 tablespoons orange liqueur

- 7 eggs, separated

- ½ cup sugar, divided

- 1 pinch salt

- Zest of one orange

Method:

1. Firstly, take a double boiler and melt dark chocolate in it.

2. Add olive oil and Orange liqueur in the melted dark chocolate.

3. Now take an electric mixture, add egg yolks and sugar in it .Beat them until the mixture becomes fluffy.

4. Then, take a different bowl. Beat egg whites with rest of the sugar and the salt until the soft peaks form.

5. Now fold the egg whites and the orange zest into the chocolate mixture.

6. Divide mousse into individual servings in small bowls and keep it in the refrigerator until servings.

7. Serve chilled and **enjoy.**

Cherry Peanut Granola

Servings: 241/4 cup s

Cook time: 1 hour

Nutrition: 250 calories

> 12 g Fat

> 4.5 g Saturated Fat

> 55 mg Sodium

> 34 g Carbohydrate

> 4 g Fiber

> 5 g Protein

Ingredients:

- 3 cups rolled oats
- ½ cup sesame seeds

- 3 tablespoons unsalted butter, melted
- ½ cup brown sugar
- 1 teaspoon vanilla
- 1 cup unsalted peanuts
- 1 cup plump unsweetened dried cherries
- 1 cup unsweetened dried coconut
- ¼ cup wheat germ
- ½ cup honey
- ¼ cup peanut oil
- ½ teaspoon cinnamon
- ½ teaspoon salt
- 1 cup dates, chopped

Method:

1. Firstly, preheat the oven to 300°F.
2. Take a large bowl and stir butter, oil, honey, vanilla and cinnamon in it. Then

add coconut, wheat germ, oil and peanuts. Toss them well for the coating.

3. Now take a non-stick baking pan spread a mixture on it. Bake it for about 30 minutes.

4. Stir it properly and place it back in the oven for about 150 minutes. Keep checking it with continues stirring for about 10 minutes until the mixture turns to golden brown.

5. Place in outside the oven and sprinkle salt over it. Now toss it in dry fruits.

6. Cool it down and put it in airtight container.

7. **Enjoy** a healthy snack for lunch box..!!

Phyllo Apple Gallette

Servings: 6

Cook time: 1 hour

Nutrition: 350 Calories

18 g Fat

2 g Saturated fat

130 mg Sodium

46 g Carbohydrates

3 g fiber

3 g Protein

Ingredients:

- 6 tablespoons olive oil

- 4 Braeburn or Gala apples, peeled, cored and coarsely chopped
- ⅓ cup dried cranberries
- 2 tablespoons brown sugar
- ½ teaspoon cinnamon
- ¼ teaspoon nutmeg
- ⅓ cup slivered almonds
- 8 (17x12-inch) sheets phyllo dough*
- 2 tablespoons powdered sugar

Method:

1. Firstly, preheat the oven to **375° F**

2. Heat 2 tablespoon olive oil over medium heat in a large skillet.

3. Mix apples, cranberries, brown sugar, cinnamon, and nutmeg in it. Cook it and stir it well for about 2 minutes.

4. Now remove it from heat, stir it in almonds and put it aside.

5. Brush 1 phyllo sheet with olive oil which should be placed in the centre of a baking sheet. Then, top with another sheet of phyllo and brush with oil. Repeat the same process with remaining oil and phyllo sheets.

6. Now, pile apple mixture in the centre of phyllo, leaving 2-3 inches from the border. Then carefully fold the sides up to form an edge around apples. Brush edges lightly with oil.

7. Bake it for about 40-50 minutes or until phyllo turns to light golden brown.

8. **Cool** it to room temperature and dust it with powdered sugar if desired.

Olive Oil Sauternes Cake

Servings: 10 pieces

Cook time: 1 hour 15 minutes

Nutrition: 280 calories

16 g fat

167 mg sodium

26 g carbohydrates

5 g protein

Ingredients:

- 5 eggs, separated, plus 2 egg whites
- ¾ cup sugar
- 1 tablespoon combined orange, lime, and lemon zest

- 1 cup flour

- ½ teaspoon salt

- ½ cup Sauternes (or other sweet white wine)

- ½ cup plus 2 tablespoons extra-virgin olive oil

Method:

1. Firstly, preheat the oven to 375 F. Now grease a 10-inch spring from a pan and line it with greased parchment paper.

2. Now, combine the egg yolks and ½ cup of the sugar, beat them until turns pale. Add the zest in a   mixture. Now fold in the flour and salt, then fold in the sauternes and olive oil.

3. Now beat the egg whites with the remaining ¼ cup of sugar until medium stiff peaks form. Then fold into the egg yolk mixture to form a smooth batter. Now pour batter into prepared pan.

4. First bake it for about 20 minutes then reduce the heat to 325 F and again bake it for 20 minutes longer, or until a toothpick inserted in the centre comes out clean.

5. Now allow the cake to cool down for about 20 minutes before unmoulding.

6. Serve and **enjoy.**

Medjool Date Truffles

Servings: 10

Cook time: 20 minutes

Nutrition: 260 Calories

        11 g Fat

        3.5 g Saturated Fat

        0 mg Sodium

        43 g Carbohydrate

        7 g fiber

Ingredients:

- 3 cups Medjool dates, pitted and chopped

- 2 shots espresso, brewed with 12 ounces water or a 12-ounce cup of strongly brewed coffee

- 1 cup pecans, finely chopped

- ½ cup shredded unsweetened coconut

- ¾ teaspoon orange or lemon zest

- 1 teaspoon ground cinnamon

- ½ cup unsweetened cocoa powder

Method:

1. Firstly, take 12 ounce of warm (not hot) coffee. Soak dates in it for about 3-5 minutes to make them soft.

2. Now drain out the dates and discard the coffee. Mash the dates with the help of a fork to form a paste on a cutting board.

3. Take a large bowl and transfer the paste to it.

4. Now take a mixing bowl and mix pecans, coconut, zest, and cinnamon in it.

5. Then, shape the paste into 1-inch balls.

6. Bring shallow bowl and put cocoa powder in it.

7. To coat, roll truffles in the cocoa powder.

8. Serve and **enjoy.**

Medjool Date Balls

Servings: 18

Cook time: 15-20 minutes

Nutrition: 155 Calories

9 g Fat

2 g Saturated Fat

2 mg Sodium

20 g Carbohydrates

3 g Fiber

3 g Protein

Ingredients:

- 1 cup raw, unsalted almonds
- 16 Medjool dates, pitted

106

- Water, for blending

- ½ cup shredded unsweetened coconut

- ⅓ cup raw unsalted almond butter or coconut butter

- 3 tablespoons cocoa powder

- 1 teaspoon cinnamon

Method:

1. Firstly, take a food processor and pulse almonds in it until coarsely ground. Place them in a bowl.

2. Now place the dates in the food processor. Pulse them until almost smooth, adding up to 3 tbs of water which will help in blending.

3. Again place almonds back to the food processor with some other ingredients such as the coconut, almond butter, cocoa powder, and cinnamon and pulse.

4. Now with the help of a wooden spoon scrap down the mixture in the food processor until all of the ingredients are completely incorporated.

5. Take a large bowl and transfer mixture in it. Now scoop mixture into 2-tbs balls rolling with your hands.

6. Carefully, place balls on a parchment-lined baking sheet.

7. Cover them and put them in the refrigerator.

8. Enjoy energy packed homemade snack.

Evoo Cake

Servings: 8

Total Cook Time: 1 hour

Nutrition: 390 Calories

22 g Total Fat

3 g Saturated Fat

450 mg Sodium

44 g Carbohydrates

1 g Fiber

5 g Protein

Instruction:

- ¾ cup extra virgin olive oil

- 1 ½ cups flour (preferably white whole wheat pastry flour)

- 2 teaspoons baking powder

- 1 cup granulated sugar

- ½ teaspoon salt

- 3 eggs

- ¼ cup milk

Method:

1. Firstly, heat up the oven to 350° F and lightly oil a loaf or cake pan.

2. Take a bowl. Mix flour, baking powder and salt in it.

3. Then, take another bowl, beat sugar and eggs in it till they become fluffy.

4. Now beat the mixture in the milk and after that in the EVOO.

5. Add few dry ingredients in it to make it dry and fold it till all that combines properly.

6. Place it in the oven for about 40 minutes and bake it until golden brown.

7. Cool it before you serve.

8. Serve and **enjoy.**

Conclusion

Thank you again for **purchasing this book!**

I hope this book was able to help you to appreciate the amazing ways that the Mediterranean diet can help you improve your overall health. You will be able to reduce your body fat levels while getting an incredible boost in everyday energy.

The next step is to take the necessary action and try all the amazing recipes.

Don't forget to consult your doctor before you start any kind of diet, especially if you have some underlying condition. All in all, I hope you enjoyed the book!

Finally, if you enjoyed this book, then I'd like to ask you for a favor, would you be kind enough to leave a review for this book on Amazon? It'd be greatly appreciated!

Click here to leave a review for this book on Amazon!

Thank you and good luck!

Other Books

- *The Ketogenic Diet for Weight Loss: Your Ultimate Guide to Rapid Weight Loss and Amazing Energy!*

- *The Ketogenic Diet Cookbook: 75+ Delicious and Healthy Recipes for Rapid Weight Loss and Amazing Energy*

- <u>The Intermittent Fasting Lifestyle: Lose Weight, Heal Your Body And Build Lean Muscle While Eating The Foods You Love: Your Ultimate Guide To Long-Lasting Weight Loss</u>

A preview of:

The Ketogenic Diet for Weight Loss: Your Ultimate Guide to Rapid Weight Loss and Amazing Energy!

Introduction

I want to thank you and congratulate you for purchasing the book, ***"Ketogenic Diet: Ketogenic Diet for Weight Loss and Amazing Energy"***.

This book contains **proven steps and strategies** on how to embark on a dietary journey that is guaranteed to revolutionize your health. In here you will discover actionable and practical information on how to lose fat and improve energy levels. If you have been on other types of diets before and have struggled to shed those pounds or even boost your energy levels, the Ketogenic diet will help you immensely.

So what is a Ketogenic diet? It is simply a diet where a person consumes foods that provide them with more fat, and very few carbs and proteins. In a Ketogenic diet, you get up to **90%** of your calories in form of fats, with the rest being split between the other two macronutrients.

The Ketogenic diet is aimed at causing a shift in the body's utilization away from glucose to fats. In other words, you are causing your body to burn fats rather than what it is normally used to – sugars. During this process, your liver produces substances known as **ketone bodies.**

A Ketogenic diet is very restrictive in terms of how many carbohydrates you are allowed to consume on a daily basis. This level is usually restricted to about **50 to 100 grams of carbs every day.** Carbohydrates have been identified as the cause of most of our society's dietary health issues. This is especially true for processed carbohydrates, which can be addictive and unhealthy. The truth is that most people aren't even aware that all those processed carbs they are eating are making them fat. **All the exercise in the world won't help you lose weight** if you are still consuming large quantities of foods laden with processed carbs. That is why the Ketogenic diet is specifically focused on minimizing the carbohydrate intake.

The quantity of fats and proteins you consume may vary somewhat, but what eventually makes a particular diet Ketogenic is the quantity of carbohydrates it contains. This may seem difficult for some people but it is precisely his measure that makes the Ketogenic diet so effective. Your body simply adapts to the new way of energy production with time. Many people have discovered that the Ketogenic diet is able to help them **burn fat and increase their energy levels** in ways that other diets had failed to achieve.

If you have never heard of or tried the Ketogenic diet, then **this book will unravel it all in a simple and clear manner.** If you already know something about this diet, then this book will still benefit you by going deeper into some of the details that are often left out in other books. You will learn the brief history of the Ketogenic diet, discover what ketone bodies and ketosis really means, and how ketogenesis impacts your body. There are also some **great recipes** that you can sample in chapter 4. In chapter 5 we discuss about the **basic principles of ketogenic diet** and we share some important points about the daily routine and food shopping. Finally, we wrap up with some of the **misconceptions and mistakes** you need to avoid.

I hope you enjoy the book!

Chapter 1: An Overview of

the Ketogenic Diet

We all know that a normal diet consist of three macronutrients – carbohydrates, proteins, and fats. The human body generally takes the carbohydrates consumed and breaks it down into glucose, which is the simplest molecule of all. Whenever glucose is detected in the bloodstream, the pancreas automatically produces insulin, a hormone that serves a very important function. Insulin will either transport the glucose to the tissues that require energy at that time, or it may trigger storage of the glucose in form of fat to be used later when required. Glucose is the obvious choice for energy production in the body because it is the simplest and easiest molecule that the body can use when energy is required.

However, a Ketogenic diet advocates for a low carbohydrate intake and elevated fat consumption. One thing to note is that going on a Ketogenic diet and fasting are somewhat similar in terms of metabolic reactions. A Ketogenic diet mimics the metabolic effects of fasting, the main difference being that you will still be consuming food. The goal here is to force your body to produce its energy and meet its calorific demands by burning fats. In order to get to understand just how this entire process works, it is critical that we look at the inner workings of your metabolism.

The moment you stop eating carbohydrates, you will experience a decline in energy reserves. This will happen quickly because your body is used to getting glucose to satisfy its fuel demands. Your body will have no choice but to look for an alternative source of energy. The next best thing would be protein. The only problem with this is that it would lead to muscle wastage, which is something you don't want. Muscles are necessary for all kinds of motion, especially when you consider things from the fight-or-flight perspective.

One viable option is **free fatty acids (FFAs).** Almost all tissues in the body, with the exception of the brain and nervous system, can use free fatty acids. In such a scenario where the body no longer relies on glucose for energy, the brain and nervous system will have to use ketone bodies as an energy source. This is what is known as ketosis. Your body will shift from burning glucose to burning ketones.

Click Here to read the full book.

Or go to the Author Page of "John T. Smith" on Amazon.

www.ingramcontent.com/pod-product-compliance
Lightning Source LLC
Chambersburg PA
CBHW062010280526
45787CB00005B/2047